How you are made

Text: Christina Palmgren

Adapted by Hilary Spiers

Illustrated by Claes and Marie-Louise Folkeson

Here is Tony with his family.
He is always asking questions.

'Where does my breakfast go, Grandpa?'
'What can I feel thumping up here in my chest, Dad?
And what are my bones for?'

'Why do I breathe Granny?
And why do I go to the toilet?'

'Why do mums and dads look different, Mum,
and when is our new baby coming?'

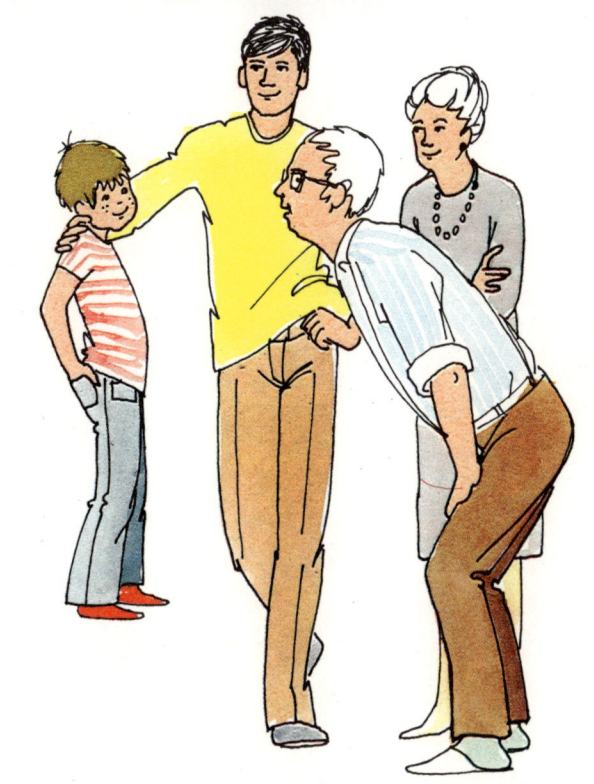

J M DENT & SONS LIMITED LONDON

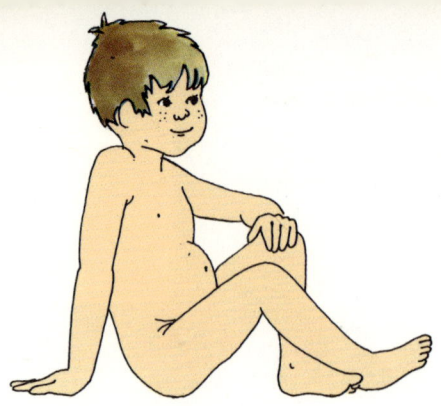

Tony's father is a man, men look like this.
Young boys look like Tony.
Between their legs at the front
men and boys have a penis.
(Lots of people call it something else.)
Some men have hair on their chest
like Tony's father.
They have hair around the penis, too,
but a boy doesn't have this hair until he is older.

All women look rather like Tony's mum.
Women look different from men.
A girl looks different from a boy
because she doesn't have a penis.
She has a small opening instead.
A woman doesn't have a penis either.
Women have breasts and a patch
of hair just like Tony's mum.
A young girl's breasts begin to grow
when she is much older,
and the patch of hair on her body
grows at the same time.

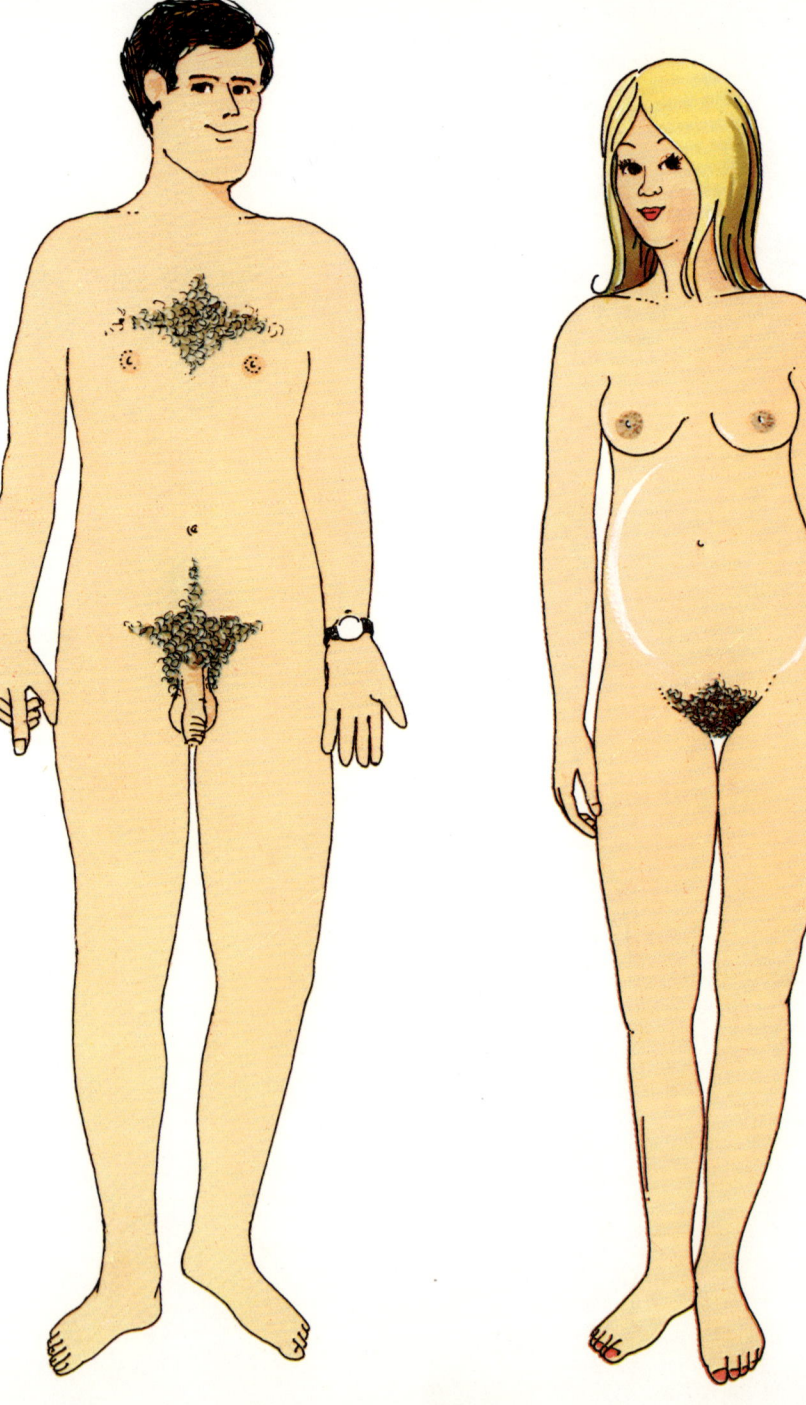

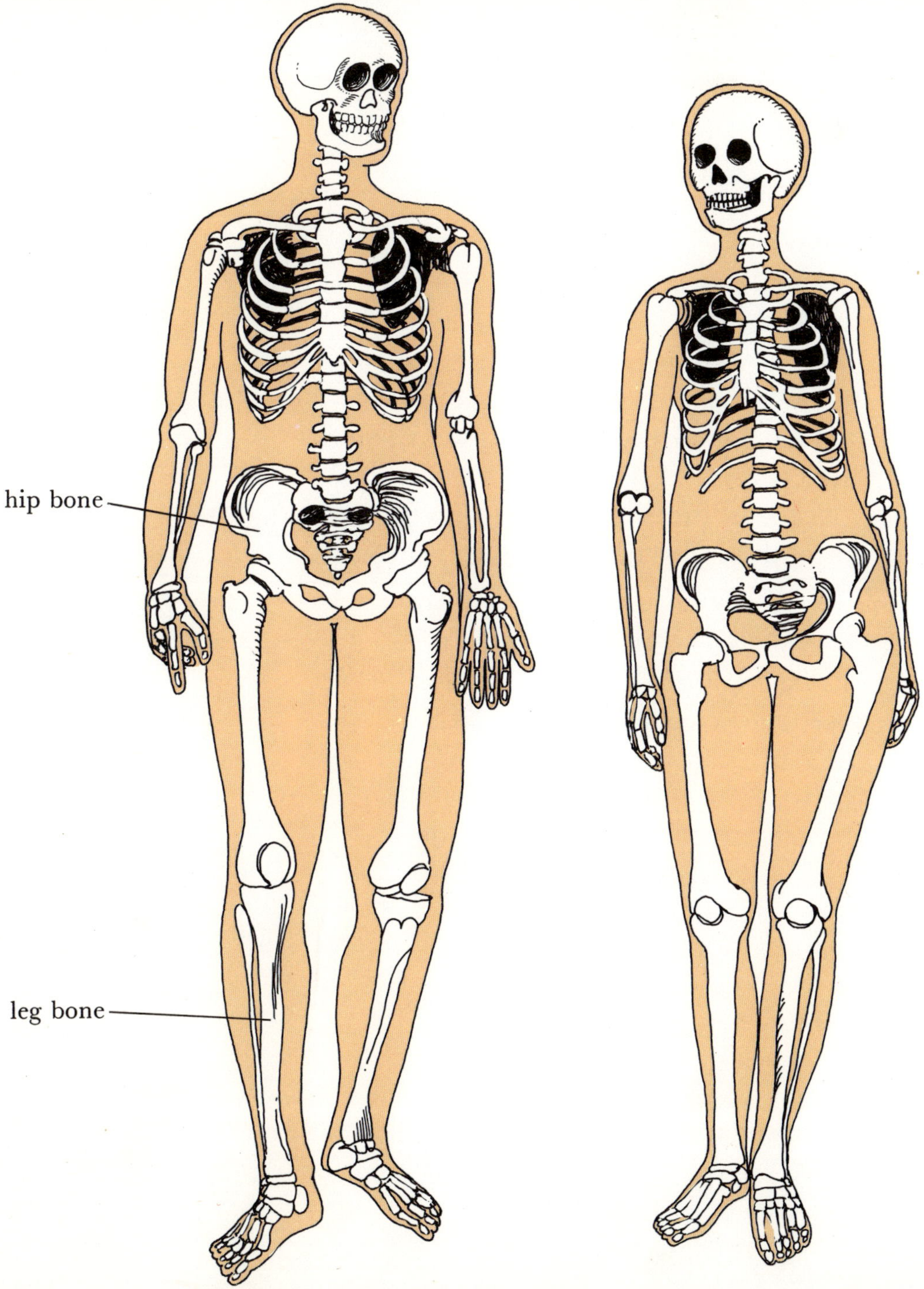

If you tap your knee or your elbow
you can feel something hard and firm.
This hardness is bone.
We have many bones inside us and they are
arranged in a pattern called a skeleton.
Your skeleton protects the
delicate parts of the body underneath
and helps you to move, too.
If you didn't have a skeleton
you would flop about and
you wouldn't be able to run
and jump and climb.
We all have skeletons which look like these.
Skeletons grow as part of us.
Your bones grow bigger as you grow older.

hip bone

leg bone

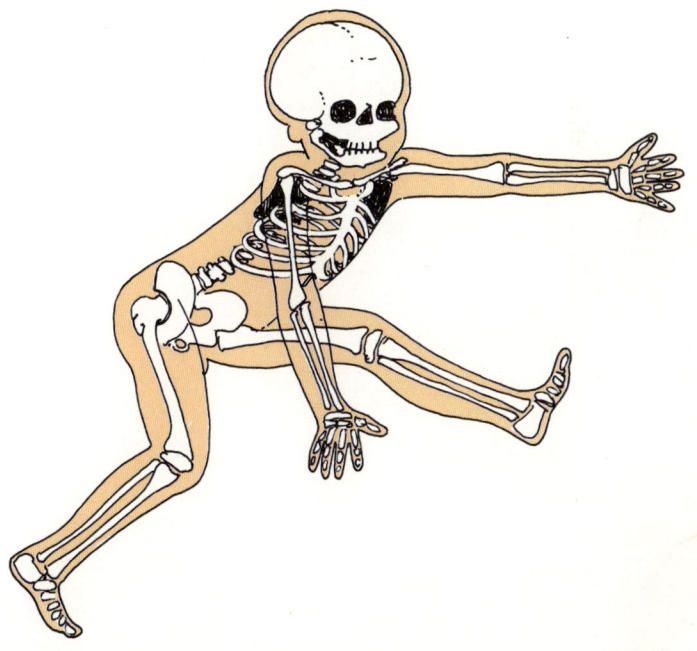

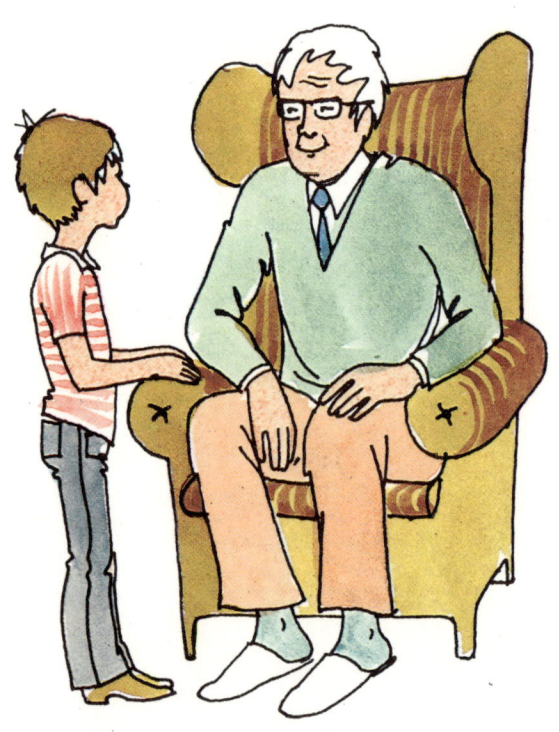

'Tell me about the thumping in my chest, Grandpa,' said Tony.
'Is that my skeleton, too?'
'No,' said Grandpa.
'We have other things inside us – delicate things
which the skeleton protects.
You have heard of your heart and your brain.
We all have these.
We need kidneys and a liver, blood vessels and two lungs,
a stomach with a long tube leading from it
called the intestine.
The human body is like a clever machine with
the different parts helping each other to work.'

Think of our muscles, for instance.
Our bones cannot move without muscles.
When you bend your arm up to your shoulder,
it is the muscle at the top of your arm
which is lifting your hand.
Muscles are attached to bones.
Muscles help you to nod your head
and touch your toes
and move your head from side to side.

Here is a picture of Tony
with his mother and father.
You will hardly recognize them.
You can see some of their muscles
around their legs and cheeks and
chins.
You can't see the bones
in their legs because
the muscles are covering them.

These strong muscles help people
to stand upright without growing
tired and to support the rest of
their heavy bodies.

You can see some of their inside
delicate parts, too.
Tony asks his family about
some of them later on.
All the parts of the body
that Grandpa mentioned
are in this picture.
Perhaps you know about
some of them already.

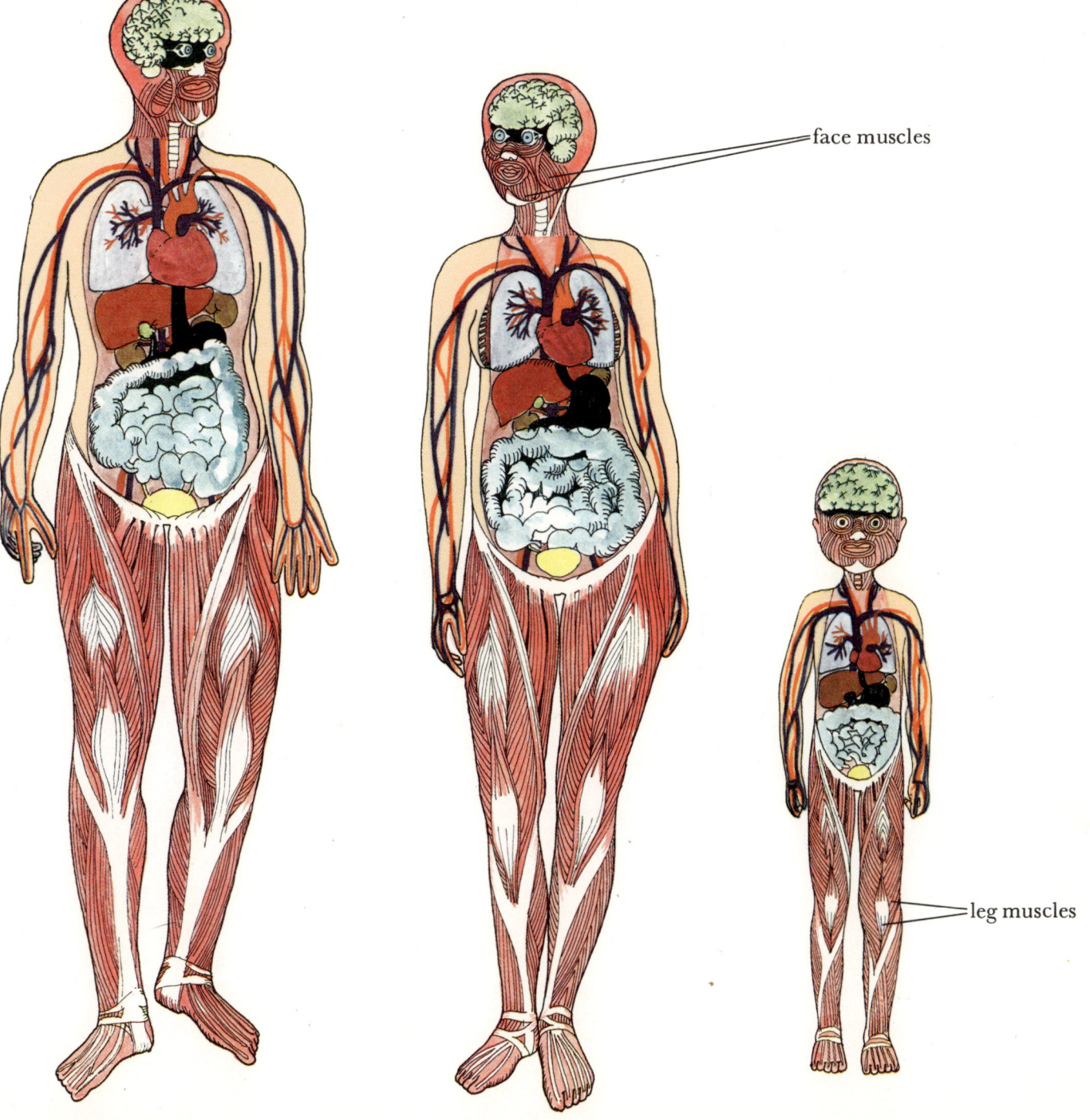

face muscles

leg muscles

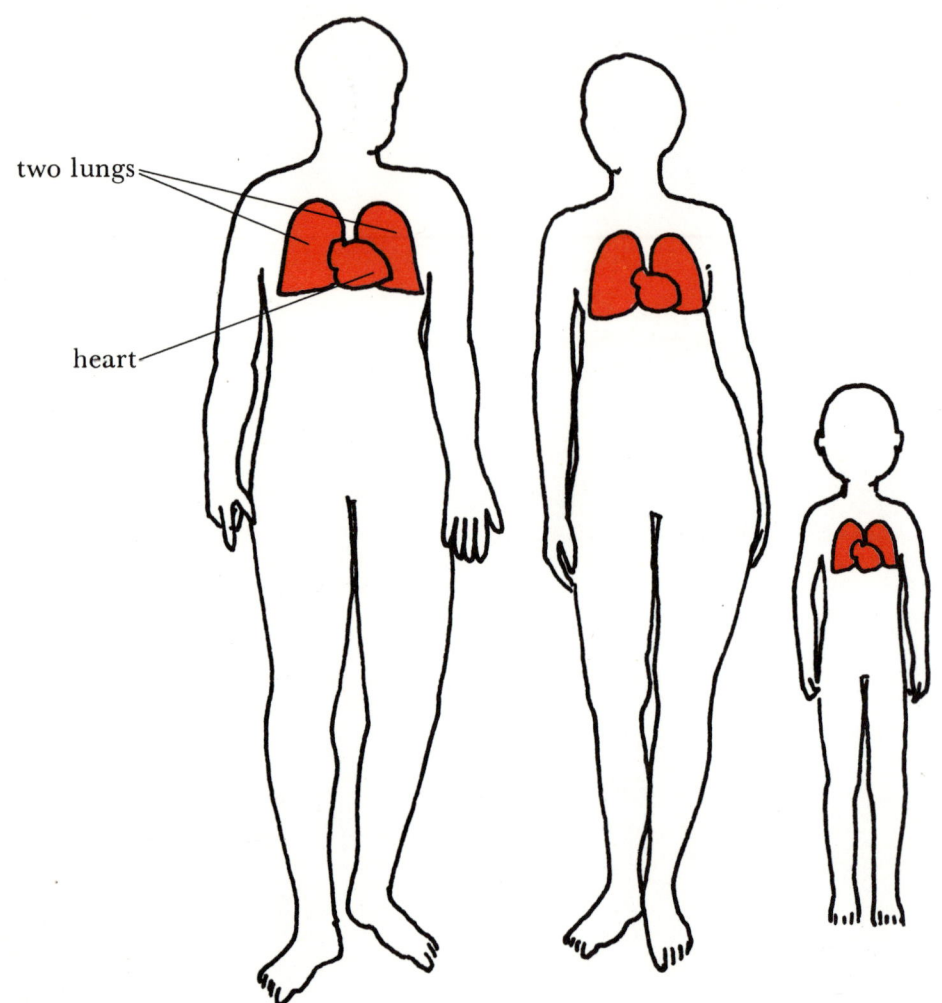

two lungs

heart

'But what about the thumping in
my chest?' Tony asked again.
'It's your heart, pumping blood around
your body,' said his mother.

'Blood travels in tubes called blood vessels.
Really, the heart is just a larger,
special blood vessel.
Blood vessels branch into smaller
and smaller vessels so that blood
can reach every part of the body.'

'Like fingers and toes?' asked Tony.
'Yes, and ears and nose,' said his mother.
'Then the smaller blood vessels join
up to make larger vessels.
These take blood back to the heart
from every part of the body.
Blood never stops. It is moving through
the blood vessels all the time.'

'But what do we need blood for?'
Tony asked.
'Blood carries important substances
which every part of the body needs.
Blood keeps the machine working,
if you like to think of it
that way,' said Grandpa.

If all the blood vessels of a
grown-up person were joined
together, they would make
a thin tube about 600 miles long.

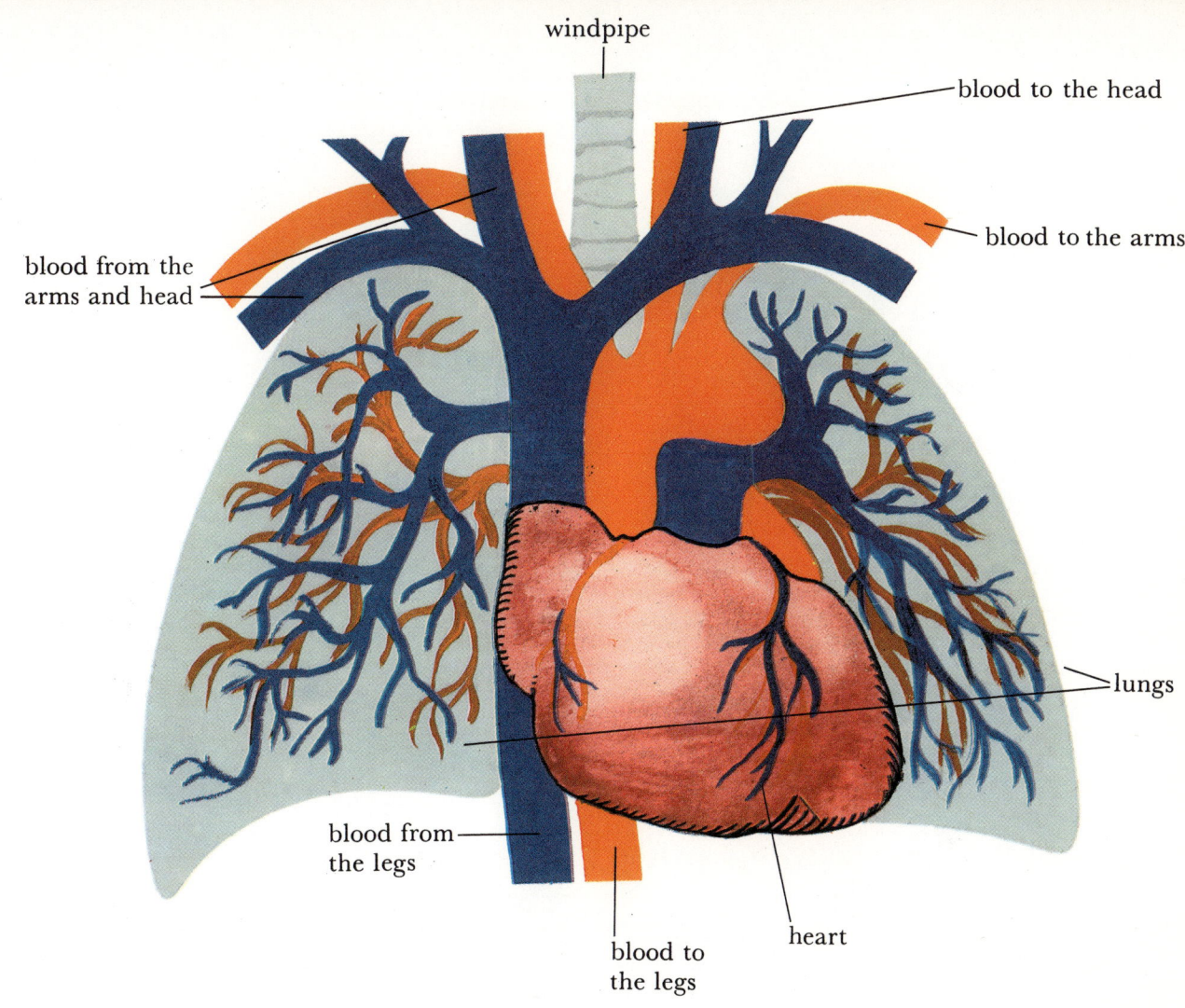

windpipe

blood to the head

blood to the arms

blood from the
arms and head

lungs

blood from
the legs

blood to
the legs

heart

'Will someone tell me about breathing?' Tony asked.

'Breathing in is taking in air through
your nose and mouth and letting the air
go down into your lungs.
You breathe air out, too.
We breathe in and out all the time, when we are
awake and when we are asleep,' said Tony's dad.

'Where is the air?' asked Tony.
'All around us. Inside the house, in buses
and cars and trains.
You can't see the air now but you can see it
coming out of people's mouths in cold weather.'

'Why do we need air inside us?' asked Tony.
'We just need the part of the air
called oxygen,' said Grandpa.
'When we breathe in, the air containing the
oxygen goes into our lungs.
The blood vessels in our lungs collect the
oxygen and then take it to the heart.
Then the heart pumps this blood with oxygen
all round the body, as we mentioned before.'

If the air around you is dirty and smoky,
it can harm your lungs.
Especially if you have your mouth open
most of the time.
The little hairs in your nose trap many of
the small pieces of dirt and dust and you can
blow them out again.
But if you breathe in through your mouth,
the dirt goes into your lungs because there
is nothing to stop it.

8

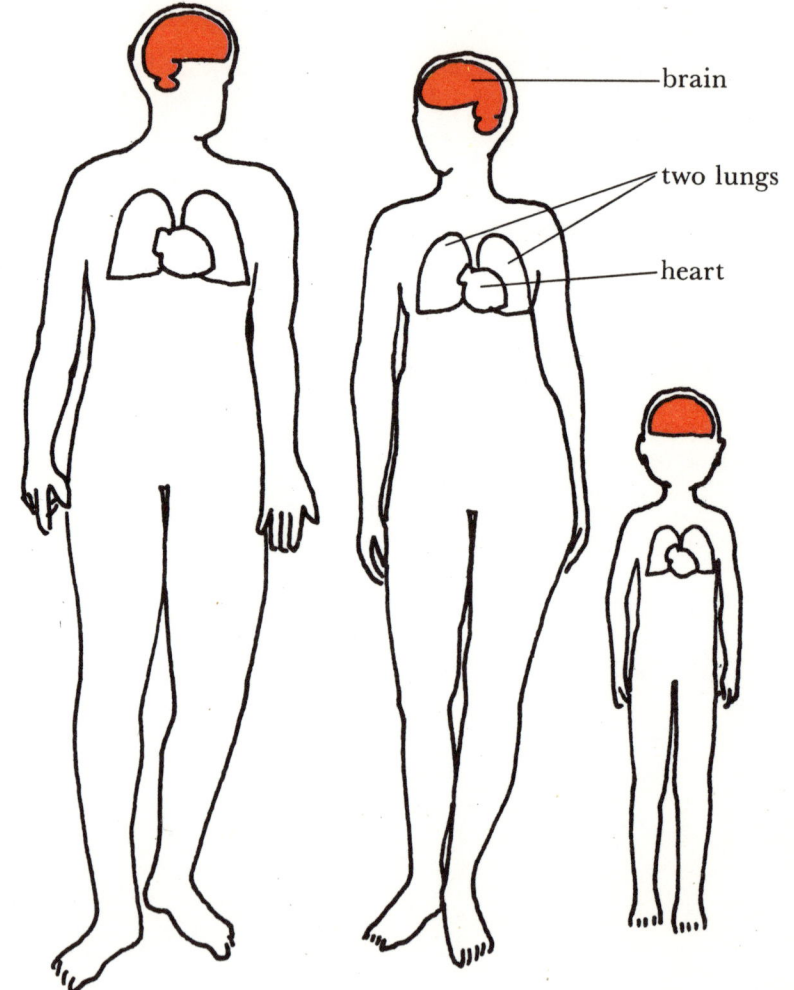

brain

two lungs

heart

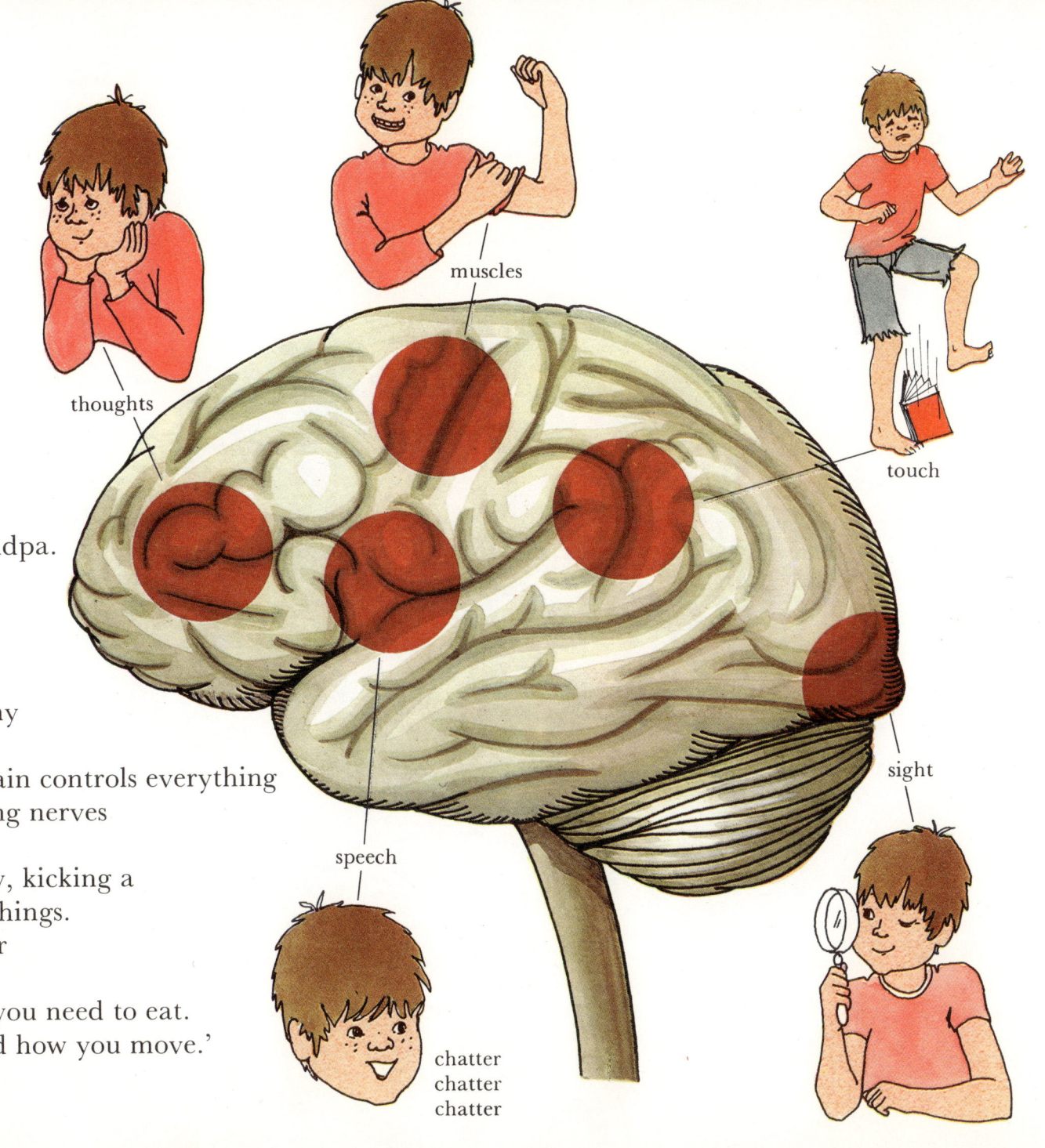

thoughts

muscles

touch

sight

speech

chatter
chatter
chatter

'What do we have brains for?'
Tony continued.
'We think with them,' said Grandpa.
'My brain thinks of lots of
exciting things,' said Tony.
'But there is more to it than
that,' said Grandpa again.
'Coming from the brain are many
string-like threads called nerves.
Without your knowing it the brain controls everything
you do by sending messages along nerves
to different parts of the body.
Pumping blood around the body, kicking a
football, seeing colours, tasting things.
The brain controls how you hear
and how you breathe.
It makes you feel hungry when you need to eat.
It controls your muscles too, and how you move.'

liver

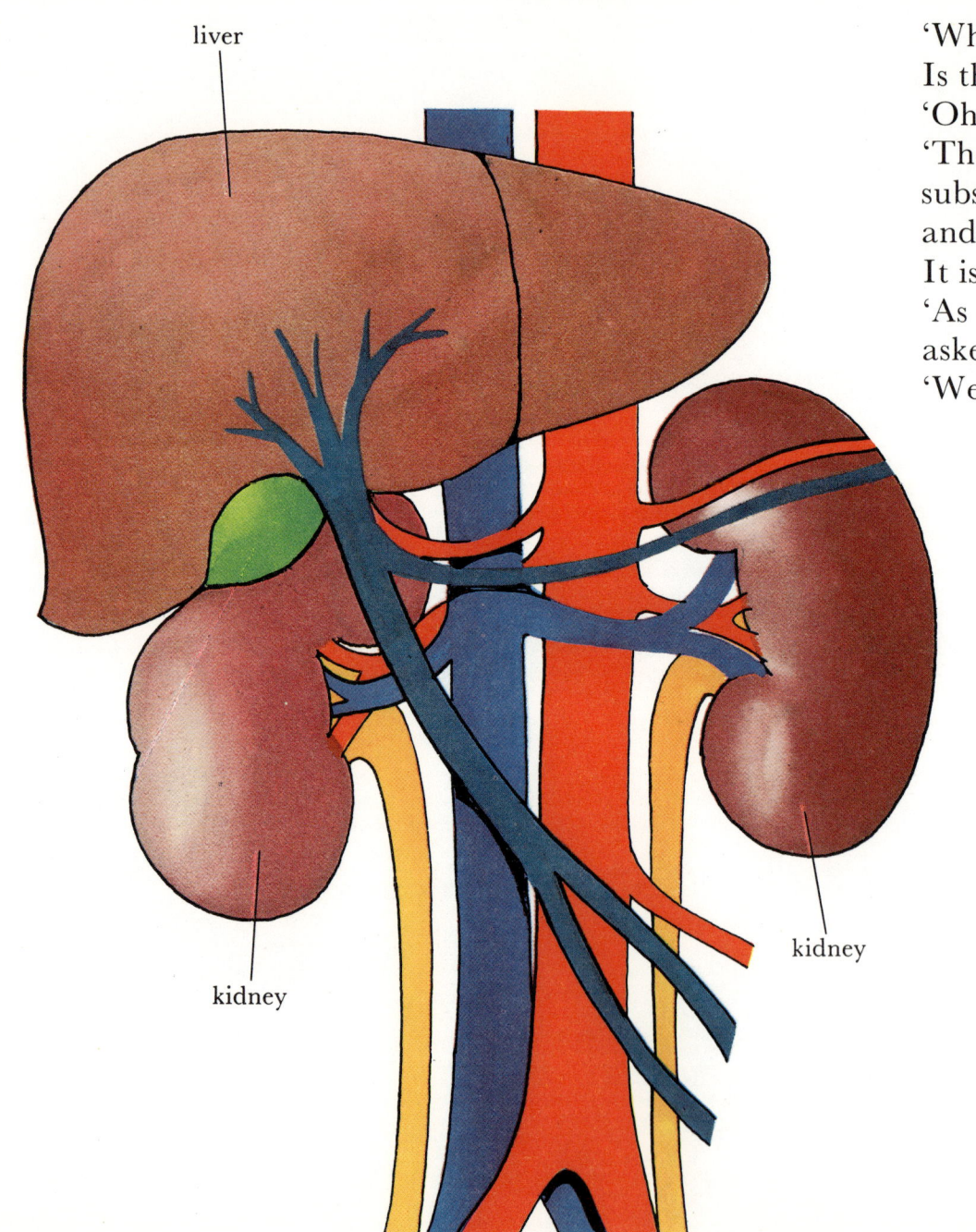

kidney

kidney

'What does my liver do?
Is that controlled by my brain, too?'
'Oh yes,' said Tony's father.
'The liver makes some of the
substances the body needs,
and it is a food store, too.
It is a very complicated part of the body.'
'As complicated as the brain?'
asked Tony.
'Well, perhaps not,' said his father.

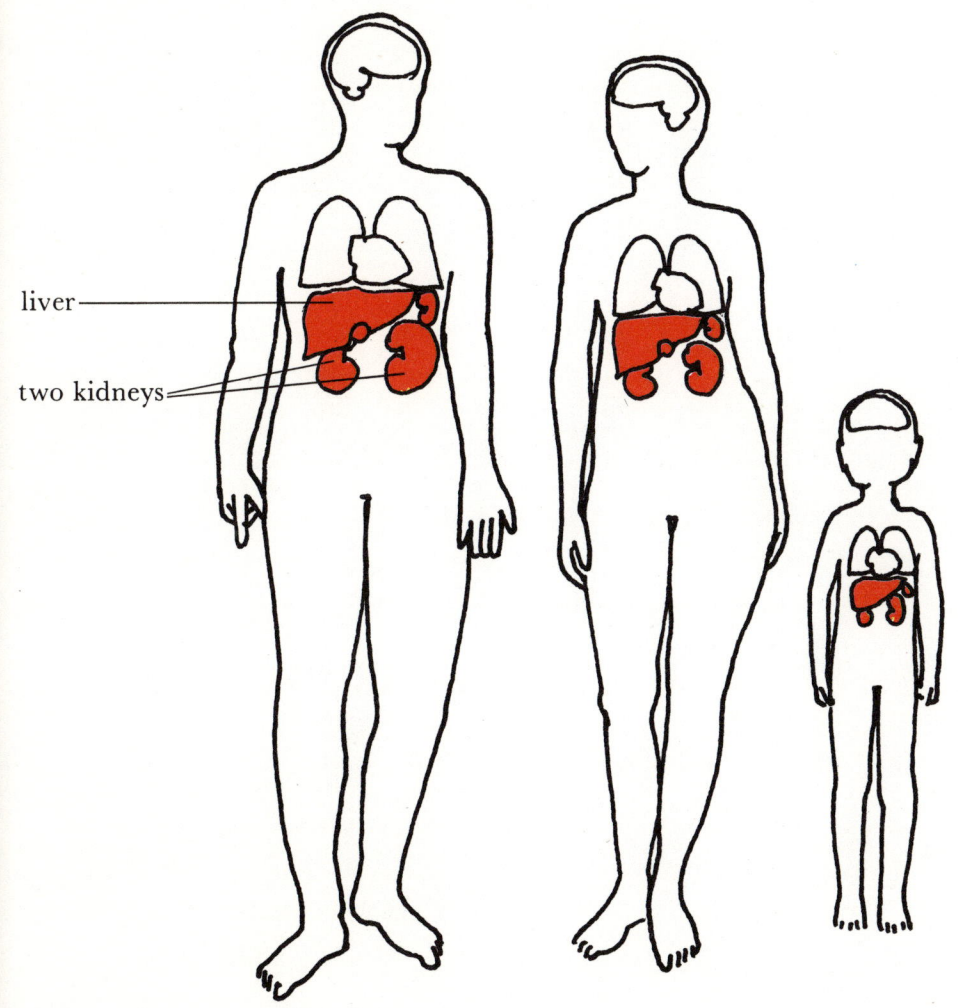

liver

two kidneys

We all have two kidneys as well.
Each kidney has two large blood vessels
to take blood to and from it.
Each kidney has another tube, called
a ureter, leading from it.

Blood takes water to your kidneys.
They keep the extra water that the body
will not need.
They send this extra water down the
ureter tubes into your bladder.
You can just see part of the bladder,
which has been coloured yellow,
in the pictures on page 5.

'When the bladder is full, the water passes
out of it down a tube passing through
your penis,' said Tony's mother.
'This is what is happening when you
go to the toilet,' she said.

'What do girls and women do Mum?'
'The water passes out of a small hole
between their legs,' said Tony's mother.

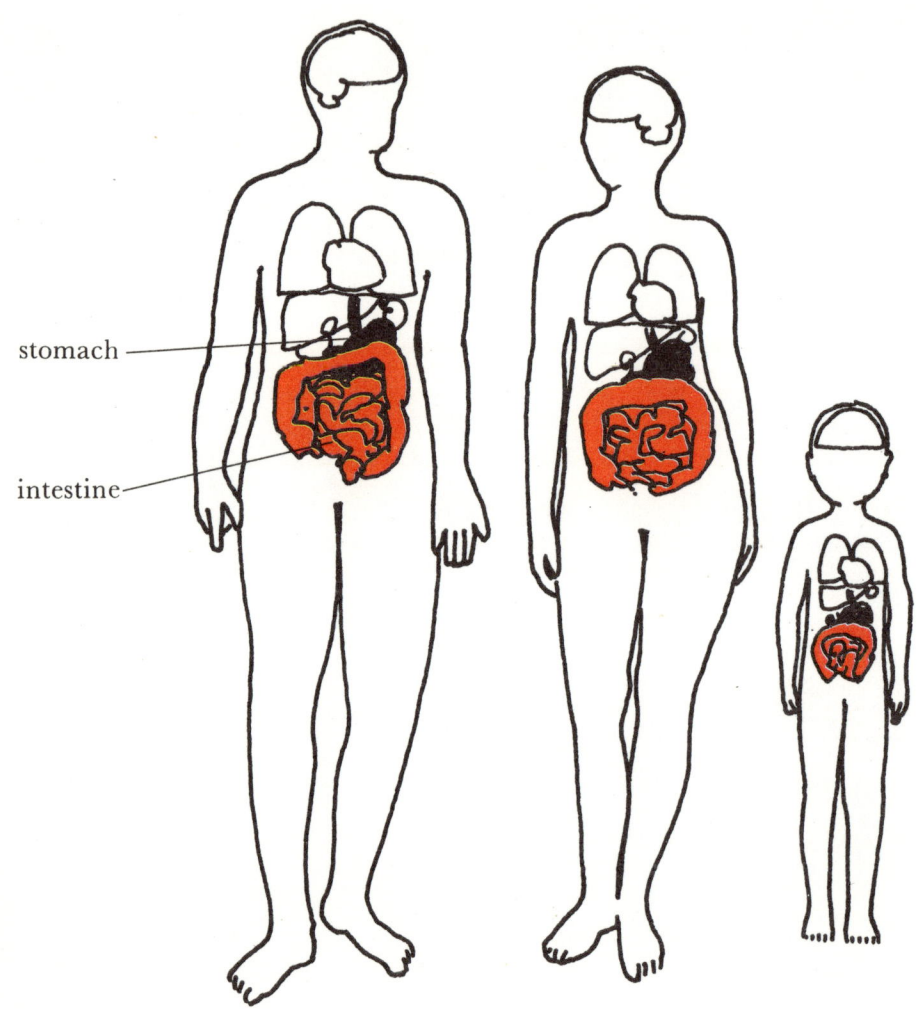

stomach

intestine

'You have told me lots of interesting things,
but you haven't said what happens to my breakfast
and my other food, too,' said Tony.

'We eat and drink because food contains many
useful substances which our bodies need,'
said Tony's father.
'Some foods help to give us energy while other
foods help us to grow and make us strong.
They help us to fight off colds and coughs
and other illnesses.'

Food has to be changed before it can give
you strength and energy.
We call this change digestion.
Your teeth start digestion by breaking
the food into small pieces.
Liquids in your mouth help too.
When you swallow, you push food down the
food pipe and into the stomach.

The stomach churns up the food and mixes it
with substances which help to change the food, too.
But it has to pass on into the long coiled tube
called the intestine before digestion
can be completed.

In the intestine, food becomes changed so that the useful parts of it can pass through into the tiny blood vessels near by. Then these useful parts of the food can be carried in the blood to the parts of the body where they are needed.

'What about the rest of the food?' asked Tony.
'The food that we don't need passes along to the end of the intestine which opens to the outside through a small hole in your bottom.
This waste food passes out of your body about once a day,' replied his mother.

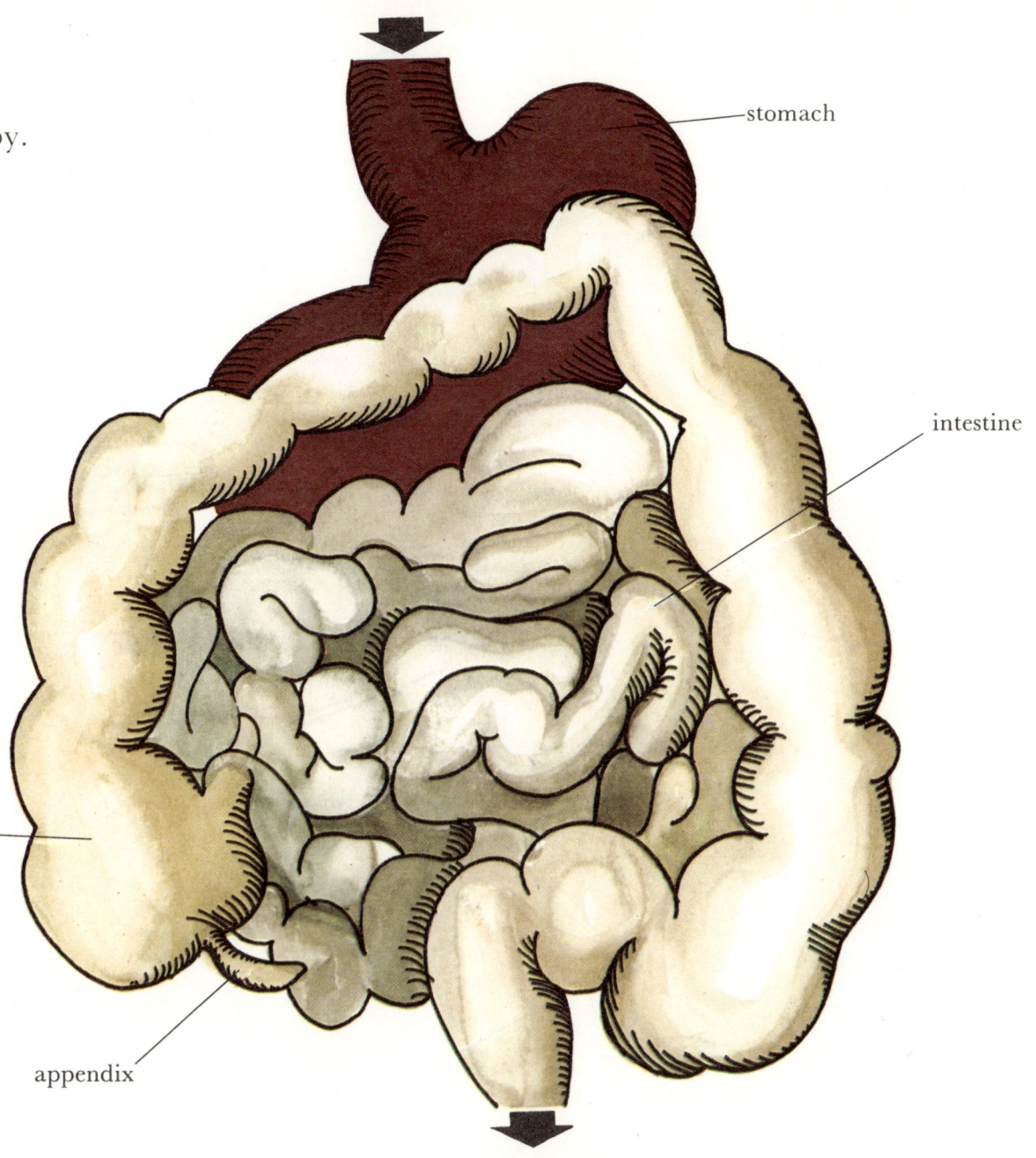

food from mouth

stomach

intestine

intestine

appendix

waste food out

13

'You haven't said anything about
the baby inside you, Mum,'
said Tony.
'How did it get there?'

'At first it was a tiny speck,
too small for you to see.
It was made just like every other
baby,' said his mother.

'A baby begins when a very, very tiny
thing called a sperm joins another
tiny thing called an egg or ovum.
After they have joined, they have become
something which will grow into a baby.
The sperm and ovum meet and join inside
the mother's body.'

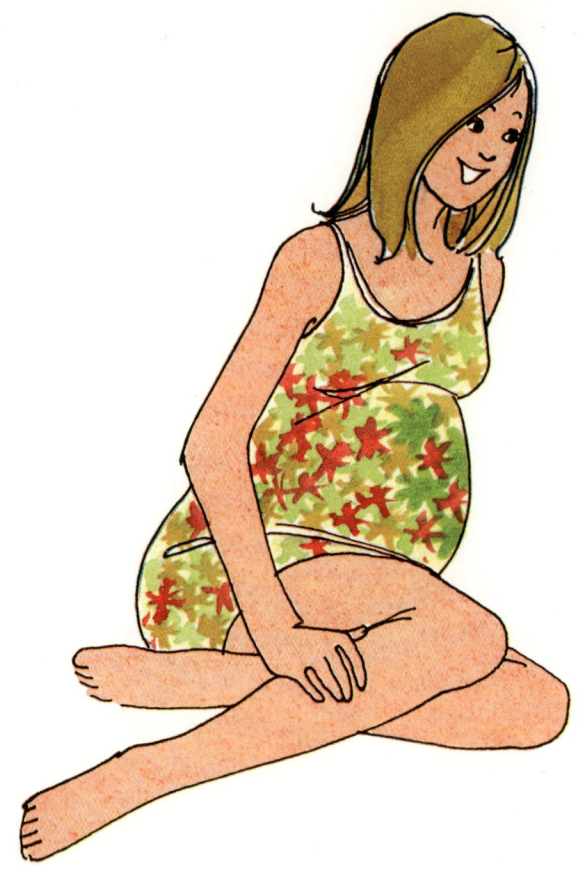

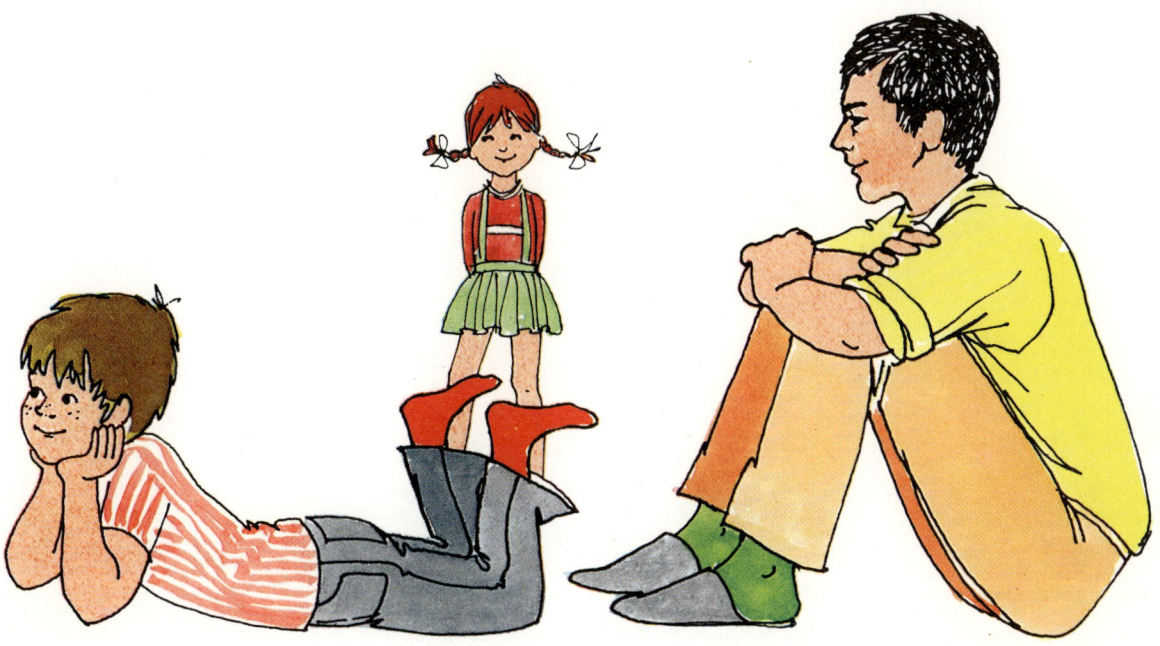

'A man has the sperm and a woman
has the ovum,' Tony's mum went on.
'There are thousands and thousands of
sperms in the bag behind his penis.'
'How do the man's sperms get into the
woman?' Tony asked.
'Through his penis,' said his mother.

All women and girls have a small hole
between their legs which leads into a
tube called a vagina.
A little girl has a very small vagina.
A woman's vagina is large enough for a
man's penis to go into it.

When a man and a woman want to have a baby
the sperms swim out of the hole at the end of
the man's penis when it is inside the woman.
One of the sperms finds its way to the ovum.
The baby can begin when the sperm has
joined the ovum.

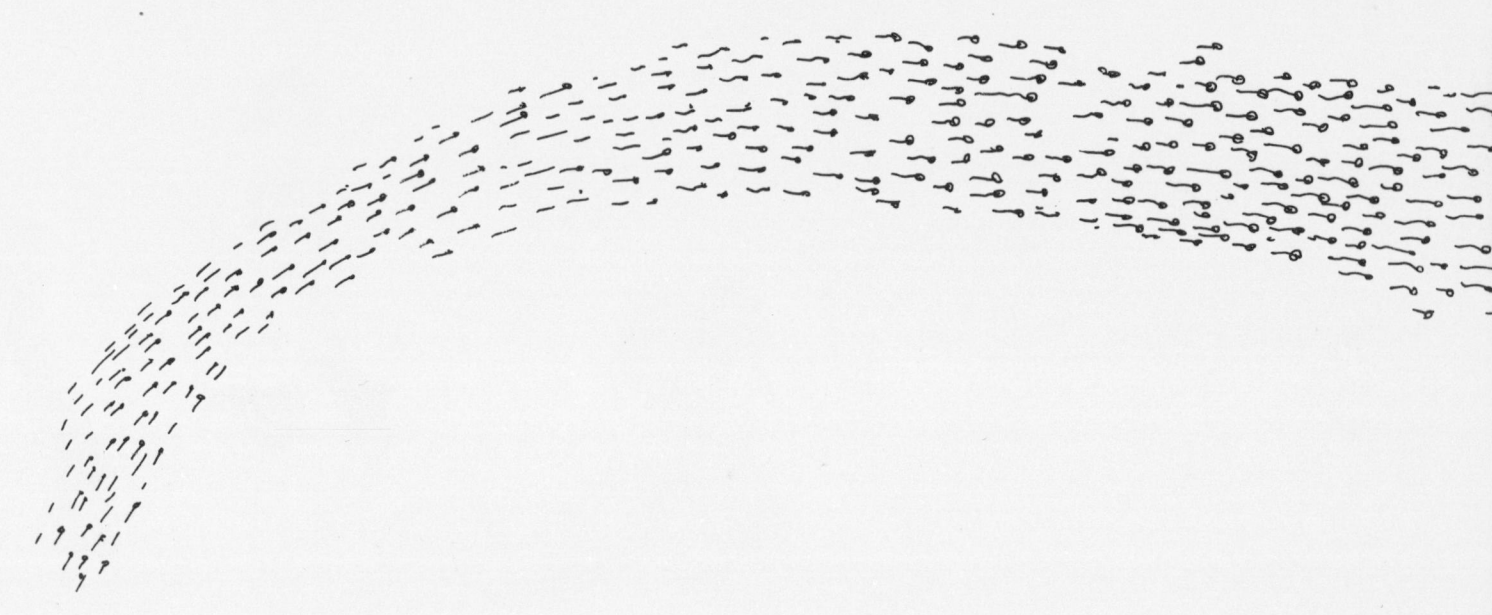

'Why are there so many sperms Dad?'
Tony asked.
'If there are lots of sperms
searching for the ovum, it is more
likely that one of them
will find it,' answered his father.

'Have you always got an ovum ready for
a baby, Mum?' asked Tony.
'No,' said his mother.
'There is only one ready for a day or two
each month.'

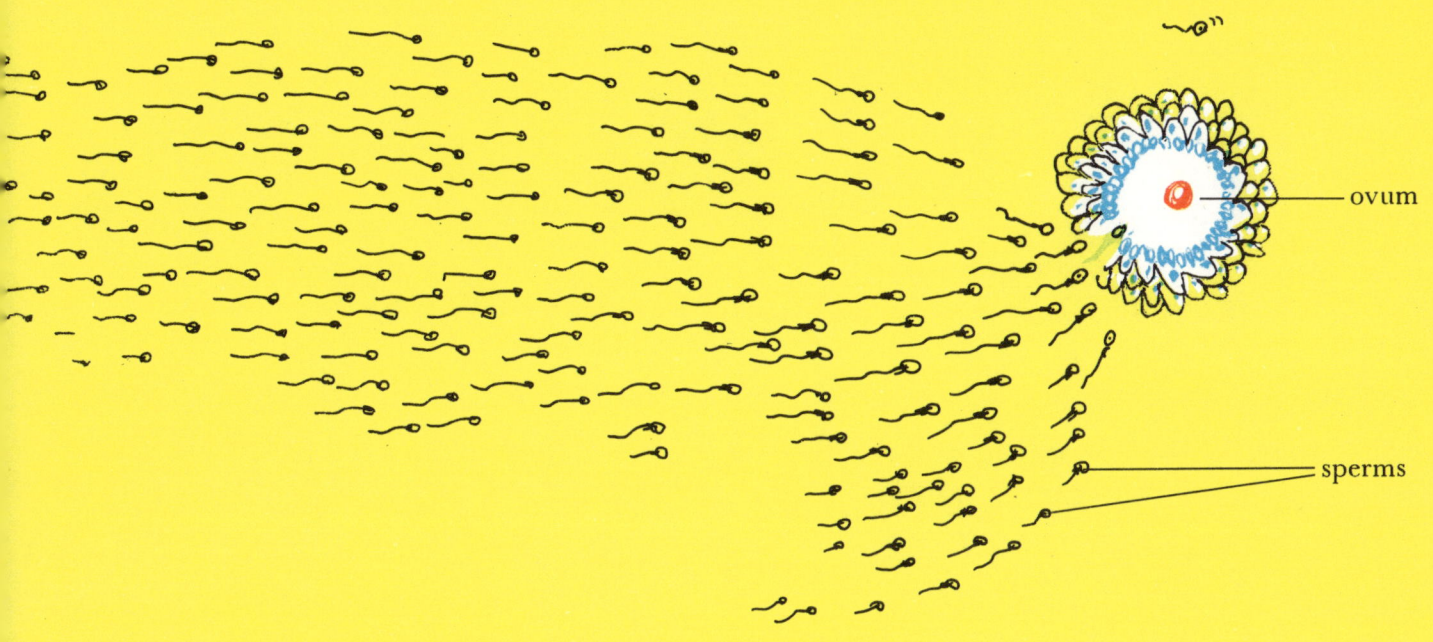

ovum

sperms

'So when you wanted me and that new baby, Dad had to be sure to put his sperms inside you then,' said Tony.

'Have I got sperms, too, Dad?' he asked.
'No, you won't start to make sperms until you are much more grown up. And it is a long time before a girl has an ovum ready, too.'

'When the sperm finds the egg does it turn straight into a new baby as small as a speck, Mum?' asked Tony.
'Oh no,' she said.
'Well how does that tiny speck become a baby?'

'When the sperm and the ovum join, they have inside
them everything that is needed to give the baby a body
and a head, and arms and legs.
They have everything that is needed to give the baby
all its inside parts, too,' said Tony's mother.

'It's all there,' said Grandpa.
'Laughter and tears, bad tempers and good tempers,
seeing and hearing, wanting to paint or play music.
All the things that we are and would like to be
come from the joined sperm and ovum.'

Soon it starts to split up into
separate compartments, called cells.
The cells grow and divide to make
still more cells, but they need food
to go on growing and dividing.
This tiny ball of cells moves to the place inside
the mother where it is going to grow into a baby,
and attaches itself to her. The place where the
baby grows is called the womb, it
gets bigger as the baby grows.

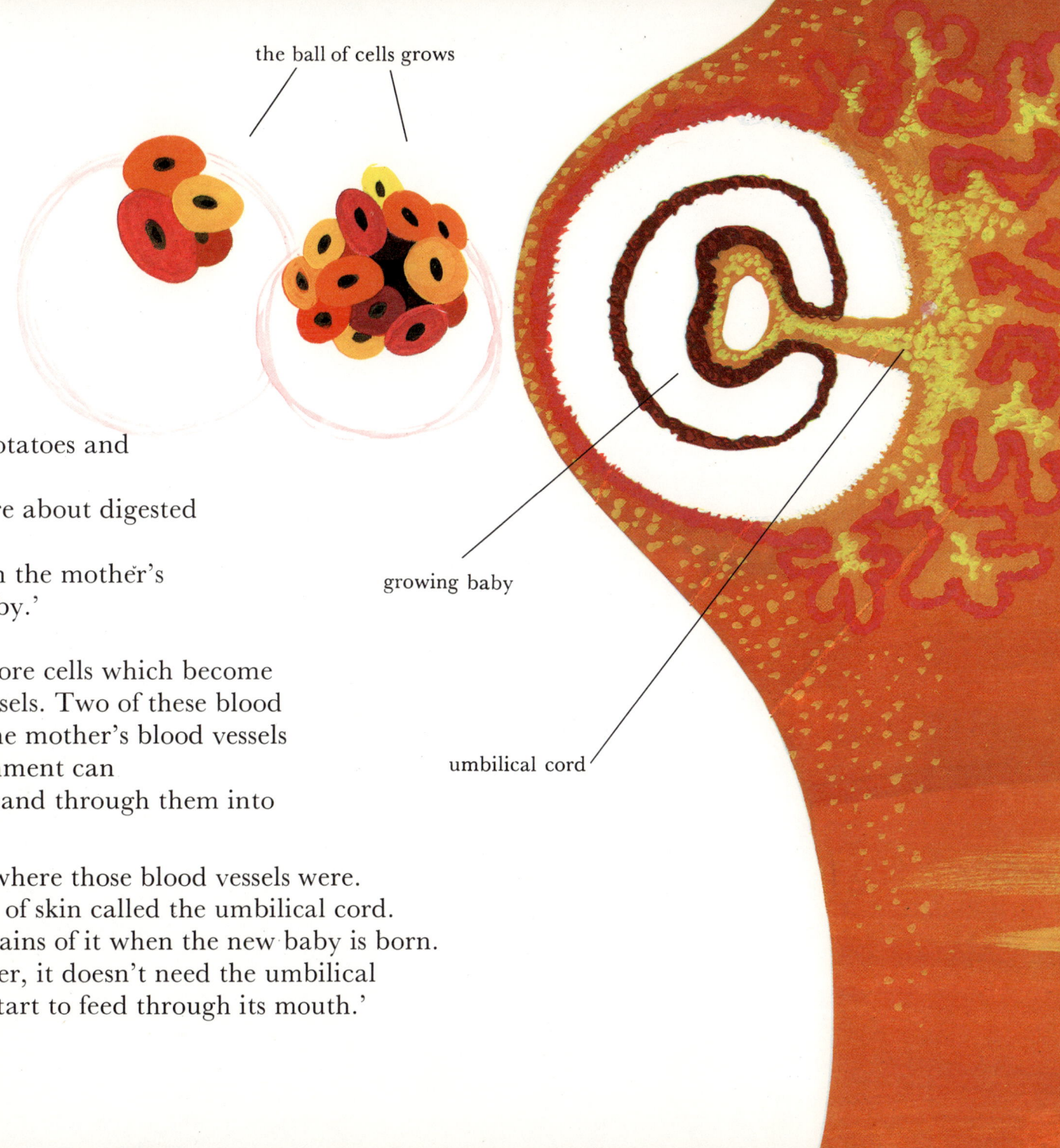

the ball of cells grows

growing baby

umbilical cord

'Does it eat things like meat, potatoes and
eggs?' asked Tony.
'Remember what we said before about digested
food, Tony,' said his mother.
'Some of the digested food from the mother's
blood passes to the growing baby.'
'How?' said Tony.
'The little ball of cells grows more cells which become
the baby's blood and blood vessels. Two of these blood
vessels grow towards some of the mother's blood vessels
in the womb. Then the nourishment can
pass into the new blood vessels and through them into
the growing ball of cells.'

'Your belly button or navel is where those blood vessels were.
They were protected by a tube of skin called the umbilical cord.
You will be able to see the remains of it when the new baby is born.
When the baby leaves its mother, it doesn't need the umbilical
cord any more because it can start to feed through its mouth.'

Actual size:

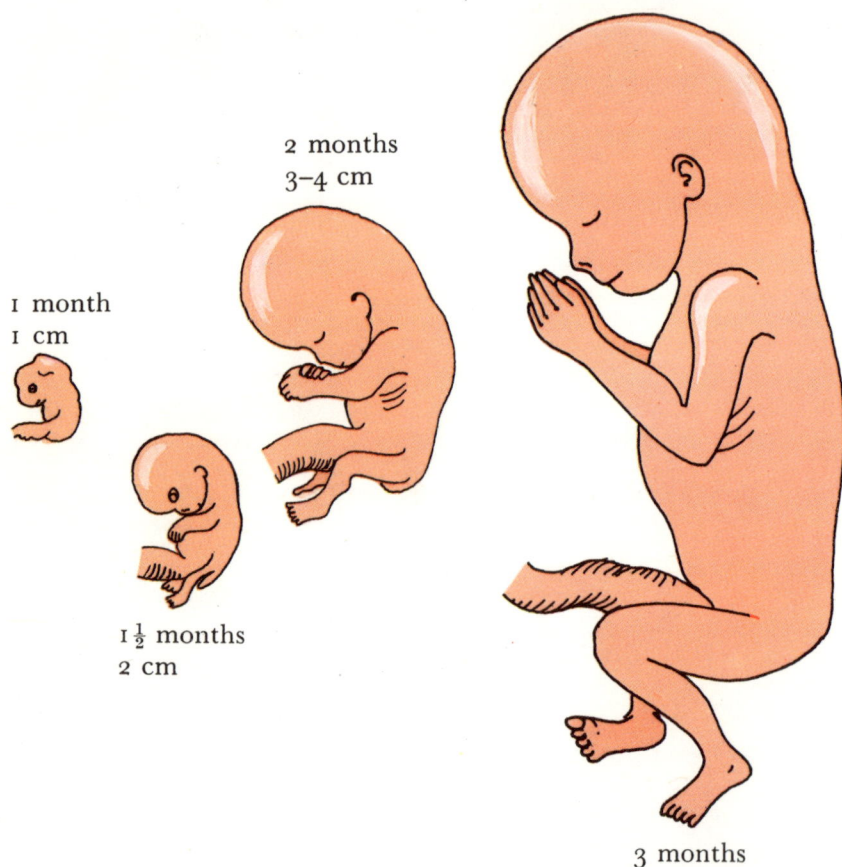

1 month
1 cm

1½ months
2 cm

2 months
3–4 cm

3 months
9 cm

Just after a baby is born the
mother's breasts begin to give milk.
Not all babies feed from their
mothers. Some have milk from a
feeding-bottle instead, and the
mother's breasts stop giving milk.

'How big was I when I had been inside
you for two months?' Tony asked his mother.
'A bit bigger than the tip of my
finger. And then after four months
you were a bit bigger than my
middle finger.
Your muscles had started to grow,
and your nose and ears, and arms
and legs, too.
And I began to feel you making
gentle movements inside me.'
'How long has the new baby been
inside you, Mum?' Tony asked.
'Eight months,' she replied.
'The baby will come out
in about a month's time.'

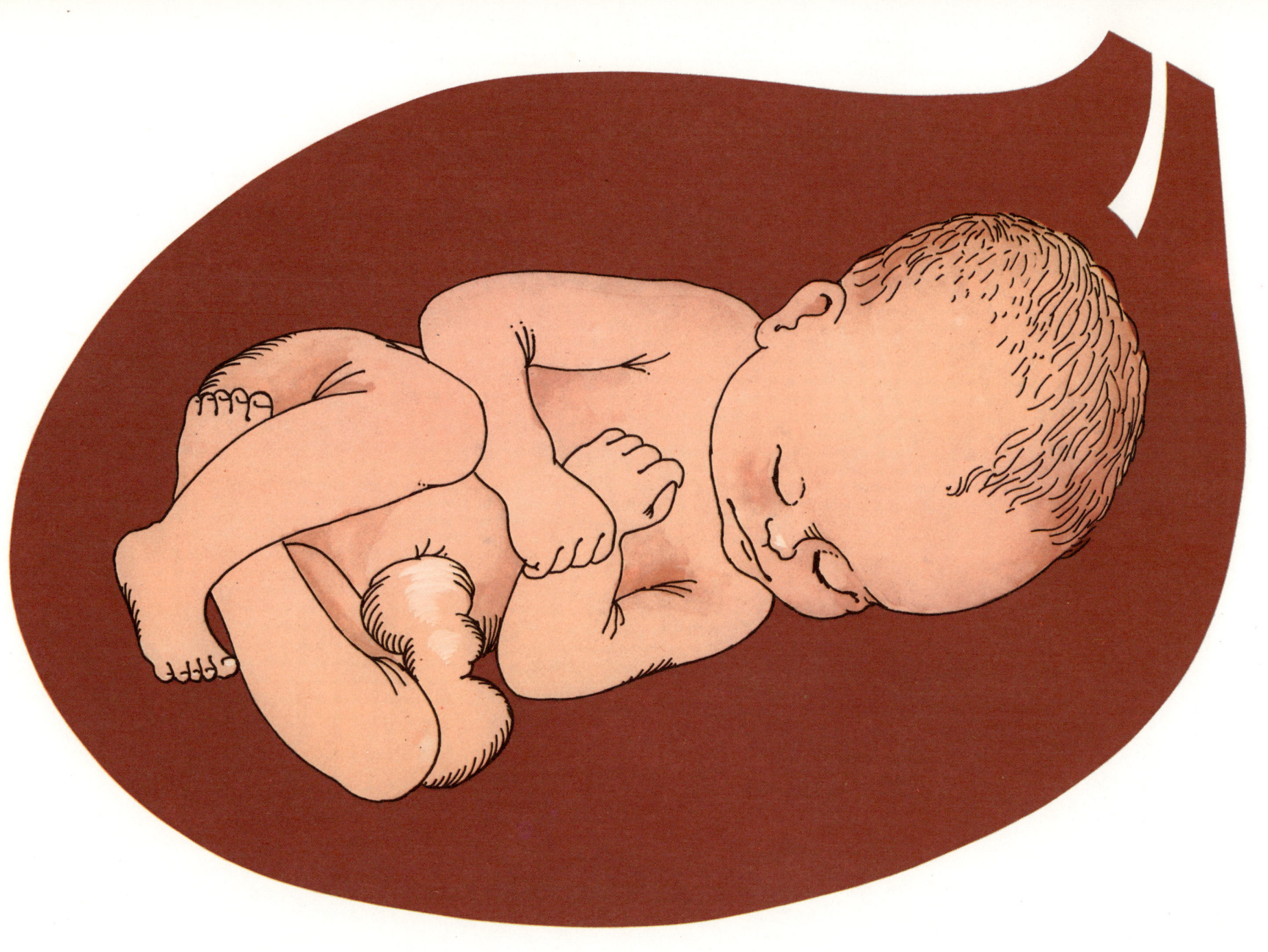

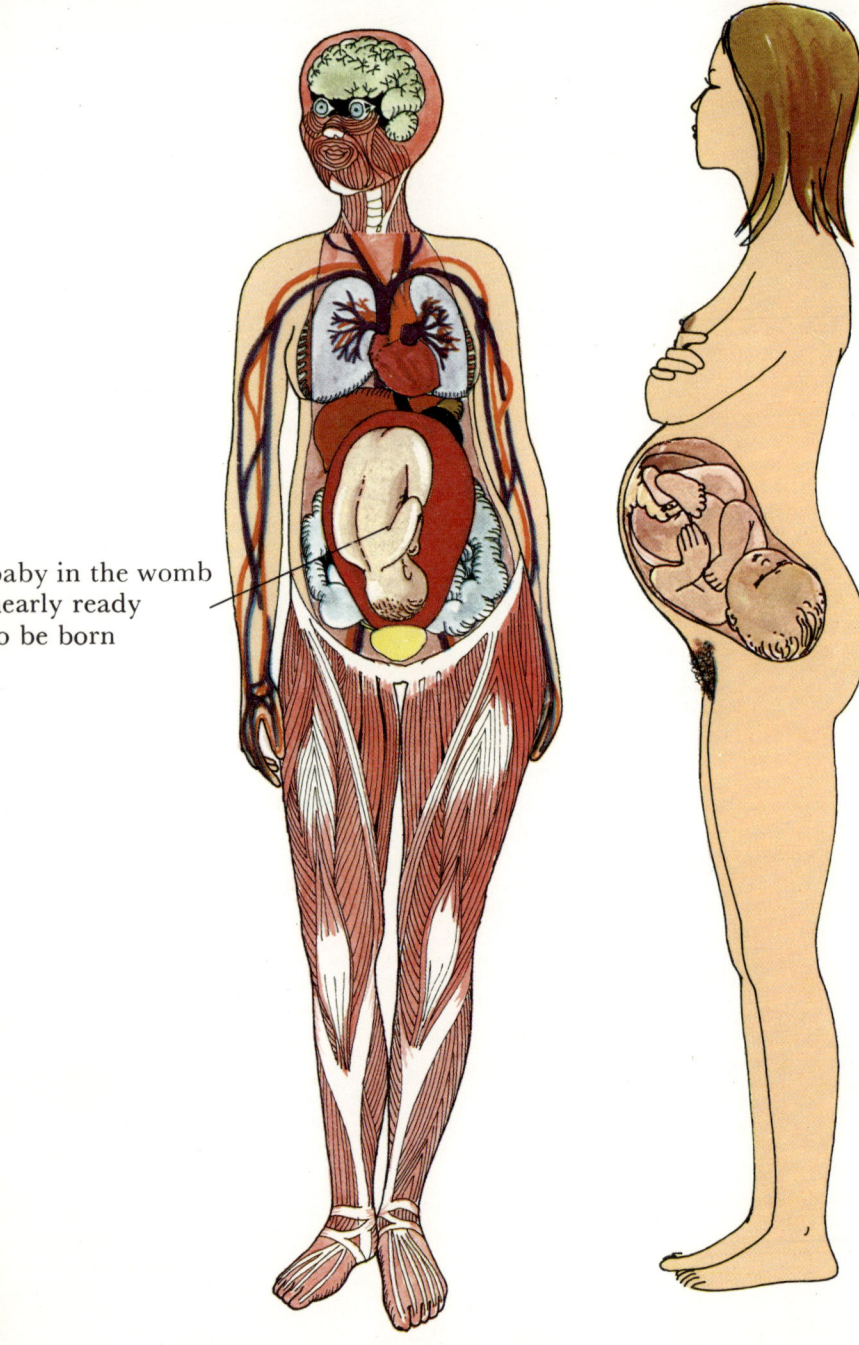

baby in the womb
nearly ready
to be born

'I hope it is a girl.'
'We can't choose, Tony, we shall have
to wait and see,' said his father.

'I wonder what the baby is like now
inside you,' said Tony.
'Well it looks like a newborn baby
curled up in there.
It has hair on its head and even
tiny finger-nails and toe-nails.
It just has to grow a bit more to
become strong enough to be born.'

'How will it get out?' Tony asked.
'Through my vagina,' said his mother.
'Now it is really only a small opening
but when the baby is ready to be born the
vagina stretches for the baby to come through.
Afterwards it becomes small again.'
'Does it hurt?' Tony asked.
'Yes,' said his mother, 'but not for long.
You soon forget all about it.'

'How marvellous,' said Tony.
'Oh yes, a baby being born is
a wonderful thing,' said his father, smiling.

remains of umbilical cord

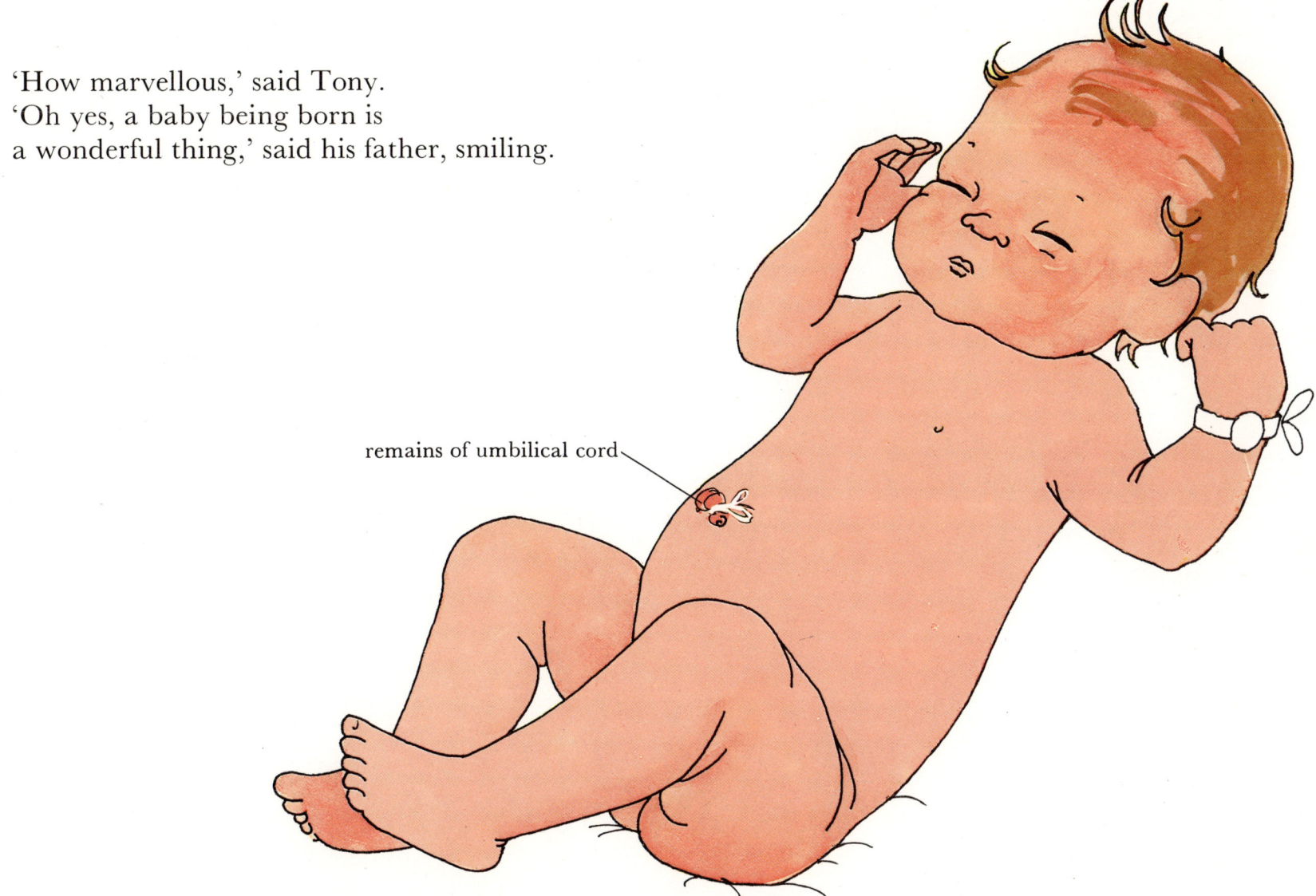

First published 1972 in Great Britain by
J M Dent & Sons Ltd, London
in Sweden by Natur och Kultur, Stockholm
in Finland by Weilin & Göös, Helsingfors
in Holland by LCG Malmberg,
's-Hertogenbosch
in West Germany by Union Verlag, Stuttgart
Medical advisor Dr Rolf Palmgren

ISBN 0 460 09567 6 Limp
ISBN 0 460 05863 0 Hardback